WONDERS OF HONEY

A step by step breakdown of simple and practical ways pure honey can be used for different benefits as well as secrets to make your honey last longer

By

Dr Henry Anderson

Copyright © 2023

TABLE OF CONTENT

CHAPTER SEVEN
BEST WAYS TO STORE RAW HONEY

CONCLUSION

INTRODUCTION

Honey is a naturally occurring sweet substance that is made by honeybees from plant nectar, plant secretions, or plant-sucking insect excretions on the living parts of plants. The bees gather this material, transform it by mixing it with specific substances, deposit it, dry it out, store it, and then allow it to ripen and mature in honeycombs.Honey is commonly utilized to make a variety of secondary products, including morning cereals, baked foods, and a wide range of other value-added commodities. It is also used as a source of sugar for honey wines and brews.

Honey is not considered a regular food in many nations; instead, it is more often used as a medication or specialty tonic. Modern medicine is beginning to recognize that honey has therapeutic benefits.

CHAPTER ONE
BENEFIT OF EATING HONEY DAILY

Eating a spoonful of honey every day can help prevent diabetes, cancer, improve heart health, and have other health advantages. Bees produce honey, which is a sticky, brown liquid that is heavily sweetened. Forage bees, often known as honey bees, gather nectar from blossoms and supplement it with enzymes.The majority of people are aware that honey is made from the nectar of flowers, but you might be surprised to learn the specifics of its production. After gathering nectar, bees ingest it and store it in a unique stomach made of honey. After that, they vomit the nectar and distribute it to other worker bees, who carry on the procedure until the honeycomb is ready for it to be applied. Honey resembles bee poop in certain ways, but it's the world's most delectable kind of vomiting.

The nectar that bees gather from flowers is used to manufacture honey; a little amount of other plant secretions and honeydew are also utilized. The flowers the bees have been feeding on determine the honey's color, scent, and consistency. Worker bees that are female are always forager honeybees. Drone bees and queen bees never go food scavenging. The foraging honey bee returns to her nest, which could be inside a man-made hive or a hollow tree or other natural hole, after visiting a flower. Her honey sac, a modified portion of her stomach, holds the nectar she extracted from the flower. Once inside the nest, she spits the liquid out and feeds it to one or more 'house' bees, who then swallow and spit it back out. Water evaporates and a tiny quantity of protein is added as each bee draws the liquid up through her proboscis and into her honey sac. The bees' additional proteins are enzymes that change the carbohydrates in the nectar into other forms. In this manner, the liquid passes throughout a network of bees before being inserted into a honeycomb cell. Bees digest the liquid in the cell once it has been placed there, evaporating more water in the process. Normally, the nest temperature in the vicinity of the honey storage area is approximately 35°C. The honey's water content continues to evaporate due to this temperature and the ventilation created by the circulating bees. The honey is deemed 'ripe' and will not ferment when the bees use a wax capping to close the cell when the water content falls below twenty percent. The bees have built up a small but well-stocked food supply for themselves, which they can keep for use in case of future flower-free periods or impending winter. The honey has been created and preserved so that there won't be any substantial quality deterioration, mold growth, or fermentation issues while in storage.

CHAPTER TWO
FORAGING BY BEES

Although they can go considerably farther, bees have been seen to forage 14.4 kilometres from their nest and frequently go five kilometres for flowers. Bees typically forage within two kilometres of their nest. The honey produced in one hive may have consequently come from flowers in an area of 12.6 square kilometers, assuming a foraging range of only two kilometers. It's fascinating and intricate how bees identify flowering plants and choose which ones to utilize for the colony. In order to meet the ever-changing needs of the colony, honeybees use a variety of strategies, such as recruiting other bees to participate in foraging, switching from collecting nectar to gathering pollen or water, deciding when to switch to new foraging sources, and making numerous other decisions about how to most effectively utilize the forage resources that are currently available.When there aren't any blooms or the weather is bad, bees use the honey they make as a food store for the colony. For instance, throughout the winter months in northern temperate regions, not many plants bloom from October to March. throughout order for bee colonies to survive during this period of reduced flowering and possibly even during the freezing temperatures, they depend on their honey stores. Bees in tropical countries must endure flower-free seasons, dry spells, and weather that prevents them from foraging, such as rain or other unfavorable conditions.

CHAPTER THREE
CHARACTERISTICS OF HONEY

One of the main ingredients in honey is glucose, which crystallizes to form granulated honey, a solid honey. Honey can be granulated naturally, and liquid honey has the same nutritional value as solid honey. The difference between liquid honey and granular honey is only in form; the process can be compared to that of ice and water. Granulation is a very common occurrence in some honeys, and practically all honey will granulate when its temperature is lowered. Similar to how various people like different types of honey, some people prefer liquid honey while others prefer granular honey. Honey can be "seeded" by adding some finely granulated honey and stirring until it is evenly distributed. This method is useful if honey is needed in the granulated state but granulates slowly. If the honey is stored at a low temperature, it will now granulate. If liquid granulated honey is needed, place the jar up to its neck in a container of warm water (60 °C) and it will quickly liquefy.But boiling honey always degrades it because it breaks down its enzymes, evaporates volatile substances, and loses flavor.

THE FOLLOWING FACTORS ARE IMPORTANT FOR RAPID GRANULATION:

- low temperature (15 °C);

- elevated glucose levels; and

- availability of nuclei (such as pollen or already-formed crystals) that can serve as seeds to initiate the crystallization process.

CHAPTER FOUR
HONEY QUALITY

Bees consistently store flawless honey, regardless of whether they live in a hive or in their own nest dug out of the wild. The quality of honey produced by bees is not affected by the environment in which they reside. Only when honey is handled by humans later on—for example, when it is collected before its water level is sufficiently high, or when it is polluted, overheated, overfiltered, or spoilt in any other way—will its quality be reduced.

CHAPTER FIVE
HOW TO CHOOSE THE RIGHT RAW HONEY

Seek for honey that is labeled as "raw" or originates from a farm that can attest to the fact that it hasn't been pasteurized. There are several types of honey available, all labeled "natural," "organic," or "pure," but none of them state that the honey is raw.

Seek out a label that expressly states "raw" and keep an eye out for any additional components, like as artificial sweeteners. You can find raw honey at health food stores, farmer's markets, and mainstream and organic supermarket stores.

CHAPTER SIX
BENEFIT OF HONEY
HONEY'S ADVANTAGES AND HEALTH BENEFITS HAVE BEEN RECOGNIZED FOR EONS.

- Beneficial for controlling weight.
- Bolsters the immunological system.
- Nourishment for your face and skin.
- Increases memory.
- Cough treatment at home.
- A homemade natural cure for dandruff.
- Utilized to treat wounds.
- Honey as an organic sedative.
- Honey has therapeutic applications.
- It's applied to burns.
- Meals are prepared using it.

USEFUL IN WEIGHT MANAGEMENT

The liver uses honey as fuel to manufacture glucose. The brain is forced to release hormones that burn fat in order to maintain high blood sugar levels due to the glucose. The majority of us have trouble losing weight because we eat too much processed food and sweets. Honey increases our body's ability to burn fat.When used appropriately, honey, a natural sweetener, can help lower cravings for other sweets and deliver a variety of vitamins, minerals, and antioxidants that can aid with weight loss.

HOW TO USE HONEY FOR WEIGHT LOSS IN FOUR WAYS

Here are four methods for using honey to help reduce weight. To enjoy these strong and delectable beverages, choose one or alternate between them as you wish.

1.How to Lose Weight by Using Honey and Water

Method: Take one glass of room temperature or lukewarm water and combine it with one tablespoon of honey. Stir thoroughly and take tiny sipfuls.

Having honey in cold water will assist offset the heat that honey produces, improving your comfort level if you have a warm body temperature or high body heat.

Additionally, honey works the same way in warm or cold water. Thus, you can enjoy warm honey water in the winter and chilly honey water in the summer with grace. There's no need to worry!

Ideal time: Early in the morning when you're not hungry.

Take care not to eat for thirty minutes after taking it.

2. How to Use Honey and Cinnamon for Weight Loss: Combine one glass of room temperature or lukewarm water with a teaspoon each of honey and cinnamon powder. Stir thoroughly and take tiny sipfuls.

Another method is to bring a glass of water to a boil with cinnamon sticks, then let it cool. Next, stir in the honey and sip.

Ideal time: Just before dinner in the evening or early in the morning when you're not hungry.

Take care not to eat for thirty minutes after taking it.

3. How to Use Ginger Juice, Lemon Juice, and Honey to Lose Weight: Pour one glass of room temperature or lukewarm water into a spoonful of honey, one teaspoon of grated ginger juice, and one teaspoon of lemon juice. Stir everything together and take tiny sipfuls.

The gut-cleansing properties of lemon, ginger, and honey combine to create an ideal concoction for boosting metabolism.

Best time: Half an hour before meals in the morning and evening.

Take care not to take it when pregnant. 30 minutes after consumption, stay away from eating.

4. How to Use Amla, Lemon, and Honey Juice for Weight Loss: Transfer one tablespoon of honey, four teaspoons of amla juice, and one teaspoon of lemon juice into a glass of room temperature or lukewarm water. Blend the ingredients together and take tiny sipfuls.

This mixture helps lower cholesterol, cleanse the stomach, and promote weight loss. Make sure the honey and amla juice are of high quality, though.

Ideal time: Only in the morning for a month when you are empty-handed.

Take care not to take it when pregnant. 30 minutes after consumption, stay away from eating.

Surely, at this point, you won't need to search for "how to use honey for weight loss?" But in addition to ingesting honey, you also need to find out what else is required to support weight loss.

STRENGTHENS IMMUNE SYSTEM

HOW RAW HONEY IS A GREAT SOURCE OF ANTIOXIDANTS AND CAN BOOST YOUR IMMUNE SYSTEM

"Phytonutrients" are naturally occurring substances that are found in food that comes from plants and have the potential to strengthen the immune system and fend against illness. Antioxidants found in honey help strengthen our immune systems. Oxidants are excessively reactive chemicals that the body releases as a result of poor diet, stress, smoking, and alcohol consumption. Free radicals can then be released as a result of these oxidants attacking healthy cells. Disease can develop if these free radicals are not controlled since they can cause damage to cells. Compounds known as antioxidants slow down or even reverse the oxidation process. At least sixteen recognized antioxidants found in raw honey seek out, target, and eliminate free radicals.

NOURISHES YOUR SKIN AND FACE

One of the natural products with the highest nutritious content is honey. It has been used in do-it-yourself skin care products and is good for your health. Honey is a popular remedy for radiant skin that stays supple, moisturized, and full-looking. Furthermore, honey's inherent enzymes make it an essential component of skin care products.

You can directly apply honey to your face. After applying it to your skin for about ten minutes in gentle circular motions, rinse it off with warm water.

13 WAYS TO USE HONEY TO NOURISH YOUR SKIN

1. Honey And Tomato For Skin

Lycopene, a carotenoid that gives tomatoes their red color, is found in them (6). According to a study, topical lycopene inhibits free radicals, which is an efficient antioxidant that can prevent cell damage.Tomatoes and honey together can maintain the health of your skin.

You'll Require

A quarter-ripe tomato
One tablespoon of unprocessed honey

Towels
Method
In a blender, puree the tomato until it's lump-free.
Well-mix the purée after adding the honey.
After using a gentle cleanser, wash your skin and
pat dry.
Put this concoction on your face. Avoid touching
the delicate skin that surrounds your eyes.
Give the mask a good fifteen minutes of wear.
Use cool water to rinse it off.
With a towel, pat dry your face.
How frequently?
Twice per week.

2. Honey And Banana For Skin

Bananas are a popular component in face masks
and are supposed to moisturize the skin. It also
makes a great foundation for any homemade face
mask. This face mask, which also contains lemon
and honey, can help keep your skin clear and stop
outbreaks.

You'll Require
One ripe banana
One tsp unrefined honey
one tsp lemon juice
Towels
Method
The banana should be mashed until lumps are
gone.

Mash the banana and mix in the lemon juice and honey.

After using a gentle cleanser, wash your skin and pat dry.

Put this concoction on your face. Be cautious not to touch the delicate skin near your eyes.

Allow the mixture to sit for ten to fifteen minutes.

Use lukewarm water to wash your face, then wipe dry with a towel.

How frequently?

Once every seven days.

3. Honey And Gram Flour (Besan) For Skin

Gram flour aids in skin exfoliation and cleansing. It also aids in lessening tanning and excessive oil. Regular usage of this face mask might help you achieve a clear complexion.

You'll Require

Two tablespoons of besan (gram flour)

One tablespoon of unprocessed honey

Water

Towel

Method

Mix the besan and honey together.

To make a smooth and uniform paste, add a little water and stir thoroughly.

After using a gentle cleanser, wash your skin and pat dry.

Put this concoction on your face. Avoid touching the delicate skin that surrounds your eyes.

Give the mixture a half-hour or so.
Use warm water to rinse the mixture.
Use a towel to pat dry.
How frequently?
Thrice every week.

4. Honey And Yogurt For Skin

L-cysteine, which is found in yogurt, has the ability to lighten skin tone. It provides a cooling and skin-soothing effect in addition to aiding in skin brightening and exfoliation. This face mask works wonders for lightening and calming sensitive skin.

You'll Require
Two teaspoons of yogurt or curd
One tablespoon of unprocessed honey
Towels
Method
In order to achieve a smooth mixture, combine the ingredients.
After using a gentle cleanser, wash your skin and pat dry.
Put this concoction on your face. Avoid touching the delicate skin that surrounds your eyes.
Give the mixture a quarter to a half hour.
Use lukewarm water to wash off the mixture.
With a towel, pat dry your face.
How frequently?
Twice per week.

5. Honey And Olive Oil For Skin

Oil cleaning is a common application for olive oil. It helps to unclog pores on the skin and eliminate dirt and pollutants from your skin when applied topically. When combined with honey, it can help maintain clear skin and stop outbreaks.

You'll Require
Two tsp honey
One tablespoon of olive oil
Towels
Method
Mix the components together until a smooth mixture is achieved.
The mixture should be microwaved for 20 seconds or so, or until just warmed through.
After using a gentle cleanser, wash your skin and pat dry.
Put this concoction on your face. Avoid touching the delicate skin that surrounds your eyes.
Give the combination five minutes or so to work.
Use a mild cleaner and lukewarm water to rinse the mixture off.
With a towel, pat dry your face.
How frequently?
Twice per week.

6. Honey And Turmeric For Skin

Honey and turmeric for radiant skin

Numerous skin disorders, including acne, can be improved by the medicinal properties of turmeric. Its antibacterial and anti-inflammatory qualities have been utilized since ancient times. This mixture can brighten your complexion, prevent breakouts of acne, and maintain clear skin. For millennia, people have used honey to lighten their skin.

You'll Require
One tsp of turmeric
One tsp unrefined honey
One tsp yogurt
Towel
Method
Mix the components together until a smooth mixture is achieved.
After using a gentle cleanser, wash your skin and pat dry.
Put this concoction on your face. Avoid touching the delicate skin that surrounds your eyes.
Give the mixture a half-hour or so.
Use a mild cleaner and lukewarm water to rinse the mixture off.
With a towel, pat dry your face.
How frequently?
Once or twice a week.

7. Honey And Rosewater For Skin

Rosewater has antibacterial properties and stops the S. aureus bacteria from growing, which is what causes acne and other skin problems.

You'll Require
Two tsp rose water
One tablespoon of honey
Towel
Method
Mix the components together until a smooth
mixture is achieved.
After using a gentle cleanser, wash your skin and
pat dry.
Put this concoction on your face. Avoid touching
the delicate skin that surrounds your eyes.
Give the mixture a quarter to a half hour.
Use a mild cleaner and lukewarm water to rinse the
mixture off.
With a towel, pat dry your face.
How frequently?
One or two times a week.

8. Honey And Sugar Scrub For Skin

The sugar and honey scrub's rough texture aids in
removing all of the dead skin cells from the surface
of your skin. This keeps the buildup off of your skin
and keeps it healthy. It would be a good idea to use
a moisturizing and nourishing face mask after the
scrub to prepare your skin to absorb moisture and
nutrients.

You'll Require
Two tsp honey

One teaspoon olive oil and three tablespoons of sugar
one tsp lemon juice
Towel

Method

Mix the components until a coarse mixture is achieved.
Use a gentle cleanser to cleanse your face.
After applying the mixture to your face, use your hands to gently scrub your skin in circular motions.
Give this a go for a few minutes.
Use warm water to wash your face, then switch to cold water.
Use a towel to pat dry.

How frequently?

Two to three times a week.

9. Honey And Coconut Oil For Skin

Psoriasis and atopic dermatitis symptoms can be relieved by extra virgin coconut oil's anti-inflammatory qualities. Honey, however, may exacerbate acne, so it's not always a good idea for oily skin types.

You'll require

One tsp finely ground virgin coconut oil
One tsp honey

Method

Combine the two components.
Give your face a 10-minute massage with the mixture.
Turn it on for a further ten minutes.

Use a light cleanser to wash your face.
Apply a moisturizer afterward.
How frequently?
Twice a week.

10. Honey And Avocado For Skin

Avocado oil is rich in linoleic and linolenic acids, along with polyunsaturated and monounsaturated fatty acids. Rat studies showed that it had excellent wound-healing abilities and could increase collagen density. Use this mask containing honey for skin repair.

You'll require
A teaspoon of avocado oil
A teaspoon of raw honey
Method
Mix the two ingredients.
Massage it on your face for 10 minutes.
Leave it for another 10 minutes.
Wash your face with a mild cleanser.
Follow up with a moisturizer.
How frequently?
Two to three times a week.

11. Honey And Oatmeal For Skin

This oatmeal and honey mixture can be used to cleanse and brighten skin. Boiling oats to make colloidal oatmeal is a great way to cleanse your skin. Its abundance of saponins aids in cleansing the skin of dirt and pollutants. By lowering inflammation, it also aids in skin calmness.

You'll Require
Boil two teaspoons of oats
One tablespoon of unprocessed honey
Method
Combine the two ingredients into a paste.
Evenly distribute it over your face.
After five minutes of massaging, let it sit for a further ten minutes.
After washing in warm water, use a light cleaner.
Apply a moisturizer next.
How frequently?
Twice per week.

12. Honey And Shea Butter For Skin

Shea butter's anti-inflammatory qualities aid in soothing and calming irritated skin. It also includes fatty acids that maintain the health of your skin, such as stearic, palmitic, linoleic, and oleic. Use this honey and shea butter mixture to hydrate your skin.

You'll Require
Shea butter, one tablespoon
One tablespoon of unrefined honey
Method
Combine the two components.
Give your face and neck a thorough massage.
Give it a good fifteen to twenty minutes.

Use warm water and a mild cleanser to wash.
How frequently?
Thrice every week.

13. Honey, Turmeric, And Sandalwood Face Pack For Skin

Sandalwood can aid with a variety of skin conditions because of its antibacterial and anti-inflammatory qualities. Hypertrophic scars, which are thick, elevated scars, can be lessened by applying sandalwood and honey, according to research. In addition to treating acne and promoting healthy skin, sandalwood oil helps soothe sensitive skin.

You'll Require
One tsp honey
One tsp of rose water or raw milk
A little spoonful of powdered sandalwood
A dash of turmeric
Method
In a bowl, combine honey with raw milk or rose water.
Include the turmeric and sandalwood powder in the mixture.
Until a smooth paste develops, thoroughly stir.
On your face and neck, apply it.
Keep it running for ten minutes.
Use warm water and a mild cleaner to rinse.
How frequently?
Once or twice a week.

BOOSTS YOUR MEMORY

3 WAYS RAW HONEY CAN HELP MEMORY AND COGNITIVE FUNCTION

1.Raw Honey Improves Gut Health

A study published in the Journal of the American College of Nutrition discovered that raw honey has significant antioxidant content as well as trace amounts of proteins, enzymes, amino acids, minerals, trace elements, vitamins, aroma compounds, and polyphenols. Oligosaccharides are a prebiotic that feeds gut flora. These nutrients serve as the body's primary source of fuel and energy, including for the brain. Since raw honey is also antibacterial, this could be an alternative. Research indicates that antbiotics can lower levels of amyloid-beta proteins, which are thought to be connected to Alzheimer's disease (they cluster into plaques that contribute to nerve cell death).

2.Raw honey's anti inflammatory qualities are known to aid digestion issues including irritable bowel syndrome (IBS). For general health and wellbeing, maintaining a balanced and healthy gut is crucial. What we consume has an impact on our gut flora, which is linked to the brain. Since the stomach is frequently referred to as the "second brain," food and the health of the gut can have an impact on our mood, memory, and cognitive abilities.

3.Another factor when considering your daily nutrition is that raw honey helps stabilize blood sugar and can reduce the risk of insulin resistance and diabetes which are linked to Alzheimer Disease and dementia. This shows that raw honey may be able to lessen the effects of these illnesses and, consequently, their detrimental effects on memory and cognitive function.

Always see a doctor first if you think you may have one of these disorders or if you are experiencing problems with your memory.

HOME REMEDY FOR COUGH

An age-old remedy for sore throats is to sip tea or warm lemon water infused with honey. However, honey by itself might also work well to suppress coughing.

In one trial, children with upper respiratory tract infections between the ages of one and five were given up to two teaspoons (10 milliliters) of honey before bed. The honey appeared to enhance sleep and lessen coughing at night.

However, you should never give honey to a child younger than one year old due to the possibility of baby botulism, an uncommon but dangerous kind of food poisoning.

Keep in mind that not all coughing is harmful. It aids in clearing your airway of mucus. Suppressing a cough is typically not necessary if you or your child is otherwise healthy.

NATURAL HOME REMEDY FOR DANDRUFF

HOW TO USE HONEY FOR DANDRUFF TREATMENT?

1. Honey and Coconut Oil to Cure Dandruff
How to use honey and coconut oil for dandruff removal?

In a 1:1 ratio, combine honey and coconut oil. Use your fingertips to gently massage the scalp after applying the mixture to the entire hair and scalp. Put on a shower hat or wrap a warm towel around your head. After 30 to 40 minutes, remove the mask from the scalp using a gentle shampoo. Twice a week, try this treatment for dandruff with honey and coconut oil.

2. Henna, Olive Oil and Honey for Dandruff Treatment

How to use henna, olive oil and honey to get rid of dandruff?

Make a paste using 3–4 tablespoons of henna powder in a basin with a little olive oil. Add one tablespoon of raw honey to the henna paste and stir to combine. Using your fingertips, gently massage the hair mask all over your scalp. After an hour, wait and wash it off with a mild shampoo. To get rid of dandruff, reapply this honey-infused hair pack once or twice a week.

3. Aloe Vera, Lemon Juice and Honey for Dandruff Treatment

How to use aloe vera, lemon juice and honey to combat dandruff?

Put two tablespoons of aloe vera gel in a bowl. Stir in 1 tbsp honey and 1 tsp fresh lemon juice. Prepare the hair mask by combining all the ingredients. After thoroughly massaging it into the scalp and hair, leave the mask on for thirty to forty minutes. Put on a shower hat to keep things tidy. Once or twice a week, repeat the process after washing it off with a light shampoo.

4. Honey and Yogurt for Dandruff Removal

How to use honey and yogurt to get rid of dandruff?

Place 4 tablespoons of fresh, plain yogurt in a bowl. Add a tsp honey to this. Combine, then apply this hair pack to the entire hair and scalp. After 20 to 30 minutes, remove it with a gentle shampoo. Once or twice a week, reapply this cure with honey to get rid of dandruff.

HOW TO USE HONEY IN HEALING WOUNDS

In honey, bacteria do not grow well. This is among the explanations for why honey is beneficial healing wounds. The honey sort of suffocates the microorganisms. There are numerous explanations for this.

There's not much moisture in honey. It doesn't have nearly as much water as the bacteria would need to flourish.
Hydroxy peroxide (H_2O_2), another ingredient in honey, aids in the fight against microorganisms. This is due to the fact that when the bees consume the nectar, an enzyme called glucose oxidase in their stomachs converts the nectar into H_2O_2 and gluconic acid, which the bees then vomit and turn into the honey that humans utilize. And honey has a high acidity. Its pH is approximately 3.9 (it can be slightly higher or lower, but it is never greater than

7.0, which is the threshold that separates basic from acidic).

HONEY AS A NATURAL SLEEPING AID

RAW HONEY, EATEN JUST BEFORE BED, HELPS YOU SNOOZE IN TWO GENERAL WAYS:

1. It gives your brain easy-to-access fuel to last all night. It replenishes the glycogen stored in your liver. Your brain receives a signal to eat when glycogen levels are low. If you go to bed having not eaten in several hours, this "hunger" may wake you up in the middle of the night and make your sleep less restful.

2. Melatonin is a hormone that your body utilizes to repair itself while you sleep, and honey helps your brain release it. The sugars in honey raise your insulin levels, which releases tryptophan, which turns into serotonin, which turns into melatonin. This is how your brain changes over time.

HOW HONEY IS USED FOR MEDICINAL PURPOSES

For thousands of years, honey has been utilized as a natural remedy for a variety of ailments. Honey has numerous medical benefits, such as boosting immunity, antioxidants, serotonin, and reducing stress and anxiety. It is also antimicrobial. Numerous medical use of honey are described in traditional medicine. The source of the flowers, the time of year, the environment, and the methods of processing all affect the composition of honey. Current studies verify that the sticky, sweet substance does, in fact, have a variety of special nutritional and therapeutic qualities. However, infants should not be given honey.

Because honey contains propolis, it has the incredible ability to destroy microorganisms. Honey has been demonstrated in studies to be effective against dozens of pathogens, including E. coli and Salmonella. One kind even combats the staph germs. Honey may cure wounds and is used to treat ulcers, bedsores, acne, and burns. The honey works better the darker it is.A teaspoon of honey will help relieve sore throats and put an end to coughing. One study found that honey eased children's coughs at night and suppressed them more effectively than two popular cough medicines.Propolis's flavonoids and polyphenols, two significant antioxidants, can be found in premium natural honey.

 Antioxidants can improve heart health by lowering blood pressure and the risk of heart attacks and strokes. Antioxidants may also improve eye health and lower certain cancer risks.

Honey may be used as a natural sleep aid because it can increase insulin levels and produce serotonin, a feel-good neurotransmitter that is turned into melatonin, a molecule that regulates sleep.

Honey has long been utilized as a calming and anxiety-relieving agent. Honey has potential calming effects.

Seasonal allergies are alleviated with honey. The raw honey from the area has the same allergens that cause people to react. A person is absorbing tiny, controllable quantities of the allergen by routinely consuming the honey. On the other hand, someone who is allergic to honey ought to stay away from it.

Honey has the ability to soothe stomach flu. Honey relieves stomach flu pain well because it reduces GI inflammation.

In addition to being high in amino acids, vitamin B6, thiamine, niacin, riboflavin, and pantothenic acid amounts that vary based on the honey's floral source and quality honey is also thought to strengthen the immune system. Furthermore, honey contains significant amounts of calcium, copper, iron, magnesium, manganese, phosphorus, potassium, sodium, and zinc.Honey is a moderate laxative and has a large number of digestive enzymes. After ingesting it, it enters the bloodstream after five hours. This helps with digestion and reduces acidity.

There is a theory that honey helps with memory. Honey's high antioxidant content helps shield brain cells from deterioration. Additionally, it aids in the body's absorption of calcium, which the brain needs in order to function and make judgments.

A tablespoon of honey contains 17 grams of carbs, making it a natural source of the food. This is the best fuel for your muscles. The body uses carbohydrates as its main fuel source, and honey can help keep muscle glycogen levels stable. This is essentially muscular energy that is saved, providing athletes with a performance boost when they need it most. In order to refuel weary muscles and energy reserves after a workout, honey can also be included in meals and snacks for exercise recovery.Because honey contains iron, copper, and manganese, it is remarkably effective at helping the body produce hemoglobin. Ancient Ayurvedic scriptures state that it aids in preserving the proper ratio of red blood cells (RBCs) to hemoglobin.

HOW HONEY IS USED ON BURN

Honey is safe for first-degree mild burns.Yes, you can use natural remedies to cure some minor burns at home, but you should first be aware of the many types of burns.

According to the National Institute of General Medical Science-Trusted Source, there are four primary burn classifications.

Burns of the first degree: The outer layer of skin somewhat reddens from these small burns, which hurt.

Burns of second degree: These induce pain, swelling, blistering, and redness, and they also impact the lower layer of skin, making them more severe than a minor burn.

Burns of the third degree: Both layers of skin may be severely damaged or destroyed by these really severe burns. These require emergency medical treatment.

Burns of the fourth degree: Not only do third-degree burns cause damage to tissue, but fourth-degree burns also penetrate fat. Once more, emergency medical care is necessary.

Apart from these four main categories, burns of the fifth degree can cause harm to your muscle and burns of the sixth degree can cause damage to your bone.

HONEY MIGHT BE SAFE TO USE ON MILD TO MODERATE BURN WOUNDS

Honey can be used to treat a superficial burn that is mild to moderate if there is enough evidence to support this. Honey contains antimicrobial, antiviral, anti-inflammatory, and antioxidant qualities, according to one reviewTrusted Source.
Make sure to get in touch with your physician or other healthcare practitioner if you have a burn that is more severe than mild.

Applying honey to wounds helps speed up healing A review of the literatureTrusted Source evaluated honey's efficacy in treating acute wounds, like burns, in comparison to other topicals and wound dressings.It was discovered that applying honey topically seemed to heal partial thickness burns more fast than using polyurethane film, paraffin gauze, sterile linen, or leaving the burn exposed.

Apply honey to a dressing to avoid a sticky mess Unless you want sticky fingers for the rest of the day, consider applying the honey to a sterile pad or gauze rather than directly on the burn. Then, place the dressing over the burn. To avoid the mess, you also can buy a medical-grade dressing that comes with honey already applied.

Honey usage involves certain precautions. "Visiting a doctor to examine the wounds and ensure there is no infection or need for surgical intervention is necessary before using medical-grade honey," One can apply honey in one of its sterile forms up to three times a day, changing the wound dressing each time, after the burn has been cleaned and properly debrided, if necessary, by a professional.

HOW HONEY IS USED TO MAKE FOOD

EASY TO ADD TO YOUR DIET

Including honey in your diet is usually simple. You can use honey in any way that you would sugar to receive a little antioxidant boost. It works great for adding sweetness to tea, coffee, or plain yogurt. It can also be used in baking and cooking.
But keep in mind that honey is a form of sugar, thus eating it will raise your blood sugar. Consuming a lot of honey, especially over an extended period of time, can cause weight gain and raise your risk of developing heart disease and type 2 diabetes.

TOP 10 THINGS YOU CAN MAKE WITH HONEY

Do you really believe that honey is just a natural way to sweeten green tea? The golden, sticky substance has numerous applications; just look past the Lipton cup. For centuries, people have consumed honey and used it in cooking, baking, medicine, and yes, drinks.

10: Honey Butter

Although honey is always a delicious delight, we suggest making honey butter at home to use as a thick topping for bread, potatoes, or veggies. It's among the simplest and most delicious things you can do with honey. (If you've ever eaten soul food or are from the South, you know what we mean.) Although it tastes great on almost everything, honey butter is typically served with starchy dishes like cornbread, biscuits, muffins, and pancakes.

The recipe is so easy to follow that it hardly merits the name. Simply mix one part honey and four parts room-temperature butter together. Use two tablespoons of honey and a stick of butter if you're only making a small quantity.Since honey's sweetness varies greatly, experiment with the ratios until you discover one that works well for you. Moreover, experiment with a small amount of cinnamon or vanilla extract for a more nuanced taste.

9: Hot Toddy

Not just tea tastes better with a few drops of honey;
there are other hot beverages as well. On a cold
winter's night, order a hot toddy for a drink that will
warm you up and please your palate. Even though
hot toddies are a popular beverage during the
colder months, it's rare to find two bartenders who
can agree on a recipe for them. Although the
definition of a hot toddy is somewhat ambiguous,
almost all recipes for the beverage combine
ingredients such as hot water or tea, honey, lemon
juice, and a little amount of brandy or whiskey.

The hot toddy is still a popular cold and flu cure,
even though the majority of doctors we know are
unlikely to recommend alcohol. It's supposed to
relieve congestion, ease sore throats, and, of
course, let you pass out. The risk is that you may
forget you're sipping hard liquor because the
cocktail's honey makes it go down so smoothly.
Thus, take it slow. You should be sick, right?

8: Challah

Legend has it that the natural sweetener we're so
fond of was used by ancient civilizations to embalm
their dead for sweet eternity. Nowadays, honey's
preservative properties help to keep baked goods
fresh, so leave the mummies in the museums and
try baking a loaf of honey challah (pronounced hah-

lah). Challah is a traditional Jewish braided loaf that's typically served with the Sabbath dinner, but it's good to snack on any time, and it makes a particularly tasty French toast.

We like our challah with honey, but there are recipes that call for sugar. If you wish to use honey instead of sugar, simply make sure you adjust the water amount so the dough doesn't get overly sticky. Before baking, brush the loaf with a glaze made from a few teaspoons of honey and egg yolk, which will give the bread a sweet and crunchy crust.

7: Sauces and Salad Dressings
Is a turkey sandwich ever complete without honey-mustard sauce? If honey barbecue sauce had never been created, would summer still be the same? Both no and no. Honey really shines in salad dressings, and sauces are its natural habitat. It's no secret that pork and honey pair nicely. Do you require evidence? Prior to roasting, try coating the pork tenderloin with a generous amount of honey. Additionally, honey is a common component of homemade barbecue sauces. The next time you fire up the grill, consider combining a few spoonfuls of honey with apple cider vinegar, Worcestershire sauce, mustard, and lemon juice to create a sweet and tangy sauce instead of utilizing store-bought barbecue sauce. To add sweetness and thicken the vinaigrette in salad dressing, consider adding a few drops of honey. Also, if the salad dressing contains

a hint of honey, your children are probably going to ask for seconds.

6: Mead

In search of a buzz? One of the first known forms of alcohol is mead, or honey wine, and it remains delicious to this day. Most wine stores have mead, but if you want to wow your friends even more, consider making a few bottles yourself.

All you actually need to make mead is some honey, unchlorinated water, wine yeast, and a fermentation bucket. That's the joy of simplicity in beer making. If you've never made mead before, you should definitely start with a smaller batch, about a gallon (3.8 liters). Online tutorials are a fantastic resource for novices. Remember that hygiene is crucial, just like it is while making beer. Sterilize buckets, tubes, and bottles, among other items you use.

5: Soups

soup with added sugar? Naturally, of course! Honey is frequently used in soups flavored with curry, ginger, or chipotle seasoning, as well as in a variety of carrot, apple, sweet potato, and squash bisques.

Naturally, it's not necessary to make it sweet though dessert soups are undoubtedly available). All it can do is add complexity and balance. Honey softens the potentially bitter flavor of the main component in soups made with parsnips or cauliflower. Spicy soups also benefit from the extra touch of sweetness that you would likely only notice if it wasn't present. For a fresh spin on a traditional winter dish, consider adding a drizzle of honey right before serving your preferred hot soup (or chili!) recipe.

4: Baked Beans

Though molasses is a common flavoring for baked beans, it's actually just one choice in this staple dish for barbecues and picnics. A great method to help sweeten baked beans and create something a little different from the usual is with honey.
Honey can introduce you to an intriguing range of flavors since it doesn't taste as strong as molasses. Many bean recipes flavored with chipotle, mesquite, rum, or bourbon call for honey, sometimes in place of molasses and sometimes in addition to it..

3: Quick Breads

A means of guaranteeing a moist banana bread? Verify that honey is called for in the recipe!
A variety of fast breads, such as those made with maize, zucchini, bananas, or beer, herbs, and cheese, can be enhanced by the sweetness and texture of honey. Not using yeast, honey imparts a subtle taste to quick-baking breads that can be quite simple to make (no kneading or waiting!).

2: Snack Bars

Honey's sticky, gooey texture makes it ideal for one specific kind of baked good: chewy, soft snack bars.

Granola bars, trail mix bars, and cereal bars are excellent honey-based goods because honey maintains its wet, sticky, and flexible quality even after baking. Making your own is a simple and healthful way to replace store-bought cereals. All you have to do is combine oats or other whole grains, honey, egg, butter, oil, and other tasty snacks you have in the kitchen. The distinct texture and sweetness of honey are well complemented by the crunch of nuts and seeds and the sharpness of dried cherries or unsweetened cranberries.

1: Cookies and Cakes

Sweets are one of the most obvious and delicious uses for honey. Honey's intense sweetness and luscious texture work very well with cookies and desserts.

Honey has a distinct flavor and is sweeter than sugar. Many recipes specifically ask for honey, rather of white sugar, as the primary sweetener; this is particularly tempting to people who prefer a more natural sweetener for their baked goods.

CHAPTER SEVEN
HOW DO I STORE RAW HONEY?

Although honey doesn't spoil quickly, there are situations where it can get contaminated. Keep honey wrapped tightly and out of direct sunlight and very hot or cold conditions.

Your honey could begin to crystallize after some time. While it can appear gritty and sweet, this is quite harmless. You can warm it just enough to melt the crystals, but be aware that cooking the honey can remove its raw qualities and turn it a darker color.

Throw discard your honey if its color has changed significantly or if it smells strange.

CONCLUSION

There is enough data to support the use of honey in the treatment of medical disorders. There must be proof that honey is used in every aspect of clinical practice. Research findings indicate that the potential therapeutic benefits of honey could stem from its antimicrobial, anti-inflammatory, apoptotic, and antioxidant characteristics. This review should give practitioners compelling data to support honey's use in medicine. More research is required to fully explore all of honey's therapeutic uses, even though several studies have already evaluated the substance's effectiveness in medical settings.

www.ingramcontent.com/pod-product-compliance
Lightning Source LLC
Chambersburg PA
CBHW071120260726
48661CB00006B/2660